Report to Congress on Mild Traumatic Brain Injury in the United States:

Steps to Prevent a Serious Public Health Problem

September 2003

The *Report to Congress on Mild Traumatic Brain Injury in the United States: Steps to Prevent a Serious Public Health Problem* is a publication of the National Center for Injury Prevention and Control, part of the Centers for Disease Control and Prevention.

Centers for Disease Control and Prevention
Julie Louise Gerberding, M.D., M.P.H.
Director

National Center for Injury Prevention and Control
Sue Binder, M.D.
Director

Suggested Citation: National Center for Injury Prevention and Control. *Report to Congress on Mild Traumatic Brain Injury in the United States: Steps to Prevent a Serious Public Health Problem.* Atlanta, GA: Centers for Disease Control and Prevention; 2003.

Dear Colleague:

Traumatic brain injury is frequently referred to as the silent epidemic because the problems that result from it (e.g., impaired memory) often are not visible. Mild traumatic brain injury (MTBI) accounts for at least 75 percent of all traumatic brain injuries in the United States. However, it is clear that the consequences of MTBI are often not mild.

In response to these concerns, Congress passed the *Children's Health Act of 2000* (Public Law 106-310), which required the Centers for Disease Control and Prevention (CDC) to submit a report to Congress on appropriate methodological strategies to obtain data on the incidence and prevalence of MTBI. To that end, CDC formed the Mild Traumatic Brain Injury Work Group, composed of brain injury experts, to determine appropriate and feasible methods for assessing the incidence and prevalence of MTBI in the United States.

This report, *Mild Traumatic Brain Injury (MTBI) in the United States: Steps to Prevent a Serious Public Health Problem*, presents the significant findings and recommendations of the members of the MTBI Work Group, which are the product of numerous discussions and a thorough review of the scientific literature. It describes the public health significance of MTBI and makes recommendations on how to better measure the magnitude of the problem of MTBI in this country. Incorporating the recommendations of this report into public health policy and public health practice will help the nation to better understand the full impact and the long-term consequences of MTBI.

Julie Louise Gerberding, M.D., M.P.H.
Director
Centers for Disease Control and Prevention
Department of Health and Human Services

Contents

Preface

In recent decades, public health and health care communities have become increasingly aware that the consequences of mild traumatic brain injury (MTBI) may not, in fact, be mild. Epidemiologic research has identified MTBI as a public health problem of large magnitude, while clinical research has provided evidence that these injuries can cause serious, lasting problems.

In response to public health concerns, Congress passed the *Children's Health Act of 2000*, which required the Centers for Disease Control and Prevention (CDC) to determine how best to measure the rate at which new cases of MTBI occur (i.e., incidence) and the proportion of the U.S. population at any given time that is experiencing the effects of a MTBI (i.e., prevalence) and to report the findings to Congress. To that end, CDC formed the Mild Traumatic Brain Injury Work Group, composed of experts in the field of brain injury, to determine appropriate and feasible methods for assessing the incidence and prevalence of MTBI in the United States.

This report presents the significant findings and recommendations of the members of the CDC MTBI Work Group, which are the product of numerous discussions and a thorough review of the scientific literature. It describes the public health significance of MTBI and recommends how to better measure the magnitude of the problem of MTBI in this country.

Executive Summary

Background

According to existing data, more than 1.5 million people experience a traumatic brain injury (TBI) each year in the United States. Of them, as many as 75 percent sustain a mild traumatic brain injury—or MTBI. These injuries may cause long-term or permanent impairments and disabilities. Many people with MTBI have difficulty returning to routine, daily activities and may be unable to return to work for many weeks or months. In addition to the human toll of these injuries, MTBI costs the nation nearly $17 billion each year.

These data, however, likely underestimate the problem of MTBI in this country—for several reasons. First, no standard definitions exist for MTBI and MTBI-related impairments and disabilities. The existing Centers for Disease Control and Prevention (CDC) definition for TBI surveillance is designed to identify cases of TBI that result in hospitalization, which tend to be more severe. MTBI is most often treated in emergency departments or in non-hospital medical settings, or it is not treated at all. Few states conduct emergency department-based surveillance, and current efforts do not capture data about persons with MTBI who receive no medical treatment. Additionally, neither hospital- nor emergency department-based data can provide estimates of the long-term consequences of MTBI.

In response to concerns about this public health problem, Congress passed the *Children's Health Act of 2000*, which required CDC to determine how best to measure the incidence (i.e., rate at which new cases of MTBI occur) and the prevalence (i.e., proportion of the U.S. population at any given time that is experiencing the effects) of MTBI and to report the findings to Congress. To that end, CDC formed the Mild Traumatic Brain Injury Work Group to determine appropriate and feasible methods for assessing the incidence and prevalence of MTBI in the United States.

The Mild Traumatic Brain Injury Work Group

The Mild Traumatic Brain Injury Work Group brought together 17 external experts from fields including epidemiology, neurology, neurosurgery, neuropsychology, statistics, and an organization representing the brain injury community. The work group was divided into two subgroups. The Definitions Subgroup developed a conceptual definition of MTBI based on clinical signs, symptoms, and neuroimaging; and an operational definition to be used in identifying cases of MTBI in administrative databases, medical records, and survey and interview results. The Methods Subgroup evaluated surveillance databases and identified those that would best capture the types of data needed to determine the full magnitude of MTBI and related impairments and disabilities.

Recommended Definitions for Mild Traumatic Brain Injury

Incident Cases of MTBI

The **conceptual definition** of MTBI is an injury to the head as a result of blunt trauma or acceleration or deceleration forces that result in one or more of the following conditions:

- Any period of observed or self-reported:
  - Transient confusion, disorientation, or impaired consciousness;
  - Dysfunction of memory around the time of injury;
  - Loss of consciousness lasting less than 30 minutes.

- Observed signs of neurological or neuropsychological dysfunction, such as:
  - Seizures acutely following injury to the head;
  - Among infants and very young children: irritability, lethargy, or vomiting following head injury;
  - Symptoms among older children and adults such as headache, dizziness, irritability, fatigue or poor concentration, when identified soon after injury, can be used to support the diagnosis of mild TBI, but cannot be used to make the diagnosis in the absence of loss of consciousness or altered consciousness. Research may provide additional guidance in this area.

Based on this conceptual definition, separate **operational definitions** of MTBI are recommended for cases identified from interviews and surveys, administrative health care data sets, and patient medical records. These operational definitions are described in detail in the **Definitions Subgroup Findings and Recommendations** section (pages 15–21).

Prevalent Cases of MTBI-Related Impairments, Functional Limitations, Disabilities, and Persistent Symptoms

The **conceptual definition** of a prevalent case of MTBI is any degree of neurological or neuropsychological impairment, functional limitation, disability, or persistent symptom attributable to an MTBI.

The **operational definition** of a prevalent case of MTBI-related impairment, functional limitation, disability, or persistent symptoms is any case in which current symptoms are reported consequent to MTBI or made worse in severity or frequency by the MTBI, or in which current limitations in functional status are reported consequent to MTBI. Symptoms and limitations are described on pages 19-21.

Recommended Methods for Mild Traumatic Brain Injury Surveillance

To obtain data on the incidence and prevalence of MTBI, established methods such as hospital emergency department- and hospital-based data collection and analysis should be the first priority. The other methods provided in this report can serve as additional sources of good information as resources and capacity will allow.

Priority Recommendations to Obtain Data on the Incidence and Prevalence of MTBI

- Increase the number of states conducting emergency department- and hospital-based TBI surveillance, and apply the recommended operational definitions of MTBI to improve detection of cases in these and national systems.

- Explore using large, national hospital discharge databases that have not been used previously for injury surveillance.

Additional Recommendations – Detection and Surveillance of New Cases of Medically-Treated MTBI

- Routinely analyze data from CDC health and medical care surveys to estimate incidence and external causes of MTBIs treated in hospital outpatient settings and those treated outside hospitals and hospital emergency departments.

- Analyze data from a collegiate sports surveillance system to assess the incidence of MTBI among participants in selected college sports.

Detection and Surveillance of New Cases (Incidence) of MTBI Not Receiving Medical Care

- Explore adding MTBI-related questions to large, existing, state-based surveys.

- Determine the feasibility of using existing, national health surveys to identify people with MTBI who do not receive medical care.

Identifying and Assessing Prevalent Cases of MTBI-Related Impairment, Functional Limitation, Disability, and Persistent Symptoms

- Explore adding MTBI-related questions to existing surveys and surveillance systems to determine the prevalence of individuals with MTBI-related functional and cognitive impairments or disabilities.

- Explore determining the occurrence of MTBI-related disabilities and impairments among children by adding MTBI-related questions to large, longitudinal studies.

- Collaborate with the Defense and Veterans Head Injury Program to use their databases to determine the occurrence of MTBI-related disabilities.

- Use existing TBI surveillance systems and registries to develop prospective follow-up studies to determine what percentage of persons with MTBI become disabled or experience persistent symptoms, and to improve linkage of brain-injury persons with appropriate services.

Establishing the Natural History of MTBI-Related Impairments and Disabilities

- Collaborate with the Defense and Veterans Brain Injury Program to use their databases to determine the natural history of MTBIs experienced by military personnel and to identify pre-existing, acute, and chronic factors that predict the likelihood of disabilities, impairments, and persistent symptoms.

- Explore adding questions to longitudinal studies to track the evolution of impairments, functional limitations, disabilities, and persistent symptoms associated with MTBI.

- Support the development of state-based TBI registries with the ability to track acute MTBI cases longitudinally.

- Develop methods to determine how pre-injury and post-injury conditions affect MTBI outcomes.

- Research how symptoms and their resolution relate to the presence of biological markers.

Documenting the Prevalence of Individuals with MTBI-Related Disabilities in Special Populations

The Methods Subgroup determined that information about special populations (e.g., persons in mental health institutions and educational settings) is not of sufficient quantity or quality to recommend MTBI surveillance methods at this time. They recommended that stakeholders coordinate activities to promote research and standardize data collection instruments and methods.

Conclusion

Evidence indicates that MTBI is a public health problem, the magnitude and impact of which are underestimated by current surveillance systems. Much research is needed to determine the full magnitude of MTBI, to identify preventable and modifiable risk factors, and to develop and test strategies to reduce MTBIs and to improve outcomes for those who sustain these injuries. Such research will inform the development of more effective primary prevention strategies and policies to address the service and rehabilitation needs of persons with MTBI. The recommendations in this report can help shape that research.

Introduction

Mild Traumatic Brain Injury:
Signs, Symptoms, and Diagnosis

Historically, clinicians and investigators have classified traumatic brain injury as mild, moderate, and severe by using the scores of the Glasgow Coma Scale, a widely-used scoring system to assess coma and impaired consciousness (Teasdale and Jennett 1974; Rimel, Giordani, Barth, et al. 1981, 1982). Patients with scores of 8 or less are classified as "severe"; scores of 9 to 12 are "moderate"; and scores of 13 to 15 are "mild."

Mild traumatic brain injury or MTBI—also called concussion, minor head injury, minor brain injury, minor head trauma, or minor TBI (Rimel, Giordani, Barth, et al. 1981; Tellier, Della Malva, Cwinn, et al. 1999; Rutherford 1989)—is one of the most common neurologic disorders (Kurtzke and Jurland 1993). It occurs when an impact or forceful motion of the head results in a brief alteration of mental status, such as confusion or disorientation, loss of memory for events immediately before or after the injury, or brief loss of consciousness. In contrast, more severe traumatic brain injuries are associated with extended periods of unconsciousness (more than 30 minutes), prolonged post-traumatic amnesia (more than 24 hours), or penetrating skull injury. Although the distinction between MTBI and more severe TBI seems straightforward, establishing definitive, measurable criteria to identify and quantify the occurrence of MTBI has proven challenging because clinicians and investigators have been using different diagnostic criteria and methodologies to study this condition (Ruff and Jurica 1999; American Congress of Rehabilitation Medicine 1993).

A variety of radiological and laboratory techniques have been used to diagnose TBI, including X-rays of the skull, computed tomography of the brain, MRI (magnetic resonance imaging), and SPECT (single photon emission computed tomography) (De Kruijk, Twijnstra and Leffers 2001; Bigler and Snyder 1995). To monitor the severity of brain damage, several biological markers, such as Serum S-100, that indicate damage to brain cells are under investigation (De Kruijk, Twijnstra and Leffers 2001; Ingebrigtsen, Romner, Marup-Jensen, et al. 2000). Although these imaging and laboratory techniques help to rule out more serious TBIs, some patients with MTBI do not present abnormalities, or the markers are not sensitive enough to accurately diagnose the condition (De Kruijk, Twijnstra and Leffers 2001; Ingebrigtsen, Romner, Marup-Jensen, et al. 2000). Thus, additional research is needed about using these and other more advanced techniques to accurately diagnose MTBI.

Consequences of Mild Traumatic Brain Injury

People with MTBI and their health care providers may fail to recognize the potential severity of a brief period of unconsciousness or memory loss caused by a blow to the head (Alexander 1995; Swift and Wilson 2001). Many individuals with MTBI do not receive medical care at the time of the injury and may later present to their primary care physician days, weeks, or even months after the injury with complaints of persistent symptoms (Alexander 1995; Kushner 1998).

A person with MTBI may manifest brief symptoms or experience persistent and disabling problems (Kushner 1998). The clinical consequences of such an injury can, for example, affect one's ability to return to work and complete routine, daily activities. In one study, employed persons who were hospitalized for MTBI lost an average of nearly four weeks of work after injury (Binder, Rohling and Larrabee 1997). Other researchers reported unemployment rates among previously employed MTBI victims of 34 percent at 3 months and 9 percent at 12 months after injury (Rimel, Giordani, Barth, et al. 1981; Guthkelch 1980). Also, people with MTBI may return to work despite incomplete recovery (Russell 1971).

Despite widespread agreement that MTBI may be associated with substantial neuro-psychological problems, there is disagreement about how often and for how long such problems persist. Some researchers suggest that pre-injury factors such as age, alcohol abuse, educational level, and neuropsychiatric history, and post-injury factors such as stress, litigation, and compensation claims may affect the recovery of persons with MTBI and contribute to their disabilities (Kibby and Long 1996). However, findings in the literature are inconsistent, possibly resulting from study design limitations (Bernstein 1999) such as the lack of a control group and the absence of a standard definition for MTBI (Culotta, Sementilli, Gerold and Watts 1996; Dikmen and Levin 1993).

Knowledge about the natural clinical history of MTBI is incomplete. Impaired attention, concentration, information processing speed, and memory are the most common, persistent complaints following MTBI; others include headaches, dizziness, nausea, fatigue, and emotional problems such as impulsiveness and mood swings (Barth, Macciocchi, Giordani, et al. 1983; Bohnen, Twijnstra and Jolles 1992; Alves, Macciocchi and Barth 1993; Macciocchi, Barth and Littlefield 1998). However, these symptoms are not specific to MTBI and commonly occur in the general population (Barsky and Borus 1999; Wessely, Nimnuan and Sharpe 1999; Iverson and McCracken 1997). Moreover, considerable variability exists in the frequency with which persons with MTBI report post-injury complaints (Steadman and Graham 1970; Rutherford, Merrett and McDonald 1978;

Alves, Macciocchi and Barth 1993; Bohnen, Twijnstra and Jolles 1992; Deb, Lyons and Koutzoukis 1998). The lack of certainty about out-comes suggests a need for follow-up studies to assess the prevalence of symptoms and disabilities in representative populations.

The Burden of All Traumatic Brain Injury in the United States

TBI, including all levels of severity, is a major cause of death and life-long disability in the United States. Each year, an estimated 1.5 million Americans sustain a TBI (Sosin, Sniezek and Thurman 1996); 50,000 die from these injuries; and 80,000 to 90,000 experience onset of long-term disability (CDC 1999). An estimated 5.3 million Americans live with a permanent TBI-related disability today (CDC 1999).

Magnitude of Mild Traumatic Brain Injury in the United States

Of the 1.5 million people who survived a TBI, 392,000 (25 percent) were hospitalized; 543,000 (35 percent) were treated in emergency departments (EDs) and released; 221,000 (14 percent) were treated in clinics and physicians' offices; and 381,000 (25 percent) did not receive medical care (Sosin, Sniezek and Thurman 1996). Of those who were hospitalized, 146,000 stayed in the hospital for only one night. These data suggest that as many as 75 percent of traumatic brain injured persons sustain mild traumatic brain injury (MTBI). Using hospital and ED data, the TBI Surveillance Program of the South Carolina Department of Health (SC DOH) identified 56,780 new cases of TBI in the state from 1996 to 2000. Of them, 86 percent (49,099) were mild injuries; of these, 85 percent were identified through ED surveillance (Table 1, page 10). Both national surveillance systems and the SC DOH data underestimate the occurrence of TBI because they do not include injured people who received medical care in other facilities, such as outpatient clinics, or those who received no medical care for their injuries.

The incidence of MTBI in EDs appears to have increased—almost doubling from 216 per 100,000 in 1991 (Sosin, Sniezek and Thurman 1996) to 392 per 100,000 in 1995–1996 (Guerrero, Thurman and Sniezek 2000). In contrast, MTBI hospitalizations appear to have declined from 130 per 100,000 to 51 per 100,000 between 1980 and 1994 (Thurman and Guerrero 1999). These findings may reflect changes in hospital practices that shift the care of persons with less severe forms of TBI from hospital inpatient care to ED and outpatient treatment. Such changes indicate a growing need to document and study MTBIs treated in EDs and outpatient settings.

**Table 1. Frequency and Distribution (Percent) of Traumatic Brain Injury
in South Carolina by Severity and Level of Care, 1996–2000**

	Level of Care		
Injury Severity	EDs Only	Hospitalization	Total
Mild TBI	41,734 (85 percent)	7,365 (15 percent)	49,099 (100 percent)
Moderate and Severe TBI	—	7,681 (100 percent)	7,681 (100 percent)
TOTAL	41,734 (74 percent)	15,046 (26 percent)	56,780 (100 percent)

Source: Selassie A. 1996–2000 South Carolina Department of
       Health Traumatic Brain Injury Surveillance Program.
       Unplublished Data.

Mild Traumatic Brain Injury: Special Considerations

We need to further explore issues related to MTBI among children and among sports participants. Very few population-based studies have examined MTBI among children (Kraus, Fife and Conroy 1987). However, existing data indicate that the rates of hospital admissions and ED visits for head injuries are several times higher among children than the general adult population (Jennett 1996), with the highest rates among children under age five (Beattie 1997) and among children in lower socioeconomic groups (Adelson and Kochanek 1998). Further research is needed to assess the magnitude of MTBI among this population and to guide prevention efforts.

Sports-related injuries accounted for 20 percent (306,000) of the 1.5 million TBIs in the United States in 1991 (Sosin, Sniezek and Thurman 1996). Of persons with sports-related TBI, 12 percent (35,000) were hospitalized; 55 percent (168,000) received out-patient care only; and 34 percent (103,000) received no medical care (Sosin, Sniezek and Thurman 1996; Thurman, Branche and Sniezek 1998). These data suggest that most sports-related traumatic brain injuries fall into the mild or moderate category. While it is important to the health of children to be physically active, we must further investigate the relationship that sports may pose on the injuries one incurs, especially if the injury occurs at a young age.

Economic Burden of Mild Traumatic Brain Injury

Max and colleagues (1991) analyzed U.S. incidence and cost data for all TBIs that resulted in hospitalization or death in 1985. MTBI accounted for $16.5 billion or 44 percent of the estimated total lifetime cost ($37.8 billion) of TBIs that year. CDC updated these estimates using incidence data from 1995 and adjusting for inflation to yield an estimated total cost of $56 billion, $16.7 billion of which was for MTBI (Thurman 2001). For several reasons, this figure underestimates the economic burden MTBI poses on the United States. First, it does not include injuries treated in EDs; this omission is significant, given the decreasing trend to hospitalize persons with TBI. Additionally, it excludes injured persons treated in other, non-hospital medical care settings, such as private physicians' offices; the costs of lost productivity and lost quality of life; and indirect costs borne by family members and friends who care for persons with MTBI. Because our knowledge about the current cost to society from TBI and MTBI is limited (Thurman 2001), these additional costs need to be quantified and need to be studied to address the impact of the changes in health care practices that shifted the care of less severe forms of TBI from inpatient care to ED and outpatient treatment and follow-up (Thurman and Guerrero 1999).

Limitations in Defining the Problem of Mild Traumatic Brain Injury in the United States

MTBI has been studied in great detail from a clinical perspective, by looking at its signs, symptoms, and management, mainly among hospitalized patients. Few studies have described the magnitude and impact of MTBI from a population perspective that includes persons who are not hospitalized (Kraus, McArthur and Silberman 1994).

Complicating efforts to establish true measures of this problem are a lack of an accepted, standard definition for MTBI; a limited understanding of the consequences of MTBI; and inadequate methods of collecting data about MTBI and its outcomes (Kraus, McArthur and Silberman 1994).

Lack of a Standard Definition

Definitions of MTBI used by clinicians and investigators vary significantly (Culotta, Sementilli, Gerold and Watts 1996; Dikmen and Levin 1993). The current CDC case definition used for TBI surveillance activities is designed to identify cases of TBI that are treated in hospitals—cases that tend to be more severe. To address this limitation, CDC recognizes a need for standard surveillance case definitions to assist in identifying new MTBI cases and cases with impairments, functional limitations, disabilities, or persistent symptoms.

Limited Understanding of Consequences of MTBI

Many health care providers fail to recognize the potential impact of MTBI (Alexander 1995; Kushner 1998; Swift and Wilson 2001). Greater awareness of the problems experienced by persons with MTBI is needed to improve recognition of the condition, to reduce the extent of MTBI-related disability, and to ensure that injured persons get the services they need to allow them to resume their societal roles.

Limitations in Surveillance

Currently, most TBI surveillance relies on hospitalization data; only a few states conduct ED-based surveillance.[1] With hospitalization rates for cases of MTBI declining and more patients with these injuries receiving care in EDs or non-hospital settings, traditional inpatient, hospital-based surveillance identifies only a small percentage of persons with MTBI. Moreover, current surveillance does not capture data about persons who receive no medical care (Thurman and Guerrero 1999).

Neither hospital discharge nor ED data can estimate the number of individuals living with the consequences of MTBI or determine the full spectrum of long-term symptoms and disabilities associated with this type of injury. Some studies have attempted to assess prognosis and sequelae of MTBI. However, because these studies were conducted in small, selected clinical samples using different methodologies, their findings cannot be generalized to the U.S. population (Dikmen and Levin 1993; Bohnen, Twijnstra and Jolles 1992).

Accurate estimates of the prevalence of MTBI-related impairments, functional limitations, disabilities, and persistent symptoms require follow-up assessments among representative samples of the brain-injured population after recovery from the acute phase of injury: for example, three months, six months, and one year or longer after injury. However, population-based studies of MTBI prevalence may have substantial limitations. For example, attrition (number of persons lost to follow-up during a study) is likely to increase as the follow-up interval increases. Also, detailed or face-to-face examinations to assess neurological impairments common after MTBI may be impractical for large, population-based samples; the amount and quality of disability-related information gathered might be limited by necessary cost-saving methods such as telephone interviewing. Research is needed to address these issues that make it difficult to estimate the prevalence of disabilities resulting from MTBI.

---

[1] CDC funds 12 states to conduct hospital discharge-based TBI surveillance and 2 states to conduct ED-based TBI surveillance.

Formation and Objectives
of the CDC
Mild Traumatic Brain Injury Work Group

To address the challenges outlined previously and to meet the objectives set by Congress in the *Children's Health Act of 2000*, CDC formed the Mild Traumatic Brain Injury (MTBI) Work Group, composed of 17 external experts from diverse fields, including epidemiology, neurology, neurosurgery, neuropsychology, statistics, and an organization representing the brain injury community. The Work Group's objectives were as follows:

- Recommend standard MTBI surveillance case definitions to help detect:

  - Persons receiving medical care for MTBI in hospitals, EDs, or other health care settings;

  - Persons experiencing MTBIs who do not receive immediate medical care;

  - Persons who experience MTBI-related impairments, functional limitations, disabilities, or persistent symptoms.

- Recommend the best ways to measure the incidence of acute cases of MTBI among persons who:

  - Receive inpatient hospital care;

  - Receive treatment in EDs or other outpatient settings;

  - Do not receive immediate medical care.

- Recommend the best ways to assess the prevalence of persons experiencing long-term impairments, functional limitations, disabilities, or persistent symptoms resulting from MTBI.

- Recommend approaches to better establish the natural clinical history of MTBI-related impairments, functional limitations, disabilities, and persistent symptoms.

- Recommend approaches to identify prevalence of MTBI-related impairments, functional limitations, disabilities, and persistent symptoms among special populations, including persons in school, special education classes, mental health institutions, and prisons.

To achieve these objectives, the Work Group was divided into the MTBI Surveillance Case Definition Subgroup (the Definitions Subgroup) and the MTBI Surveillance Methods and Database Subgroup (the Methods Subgroup). As a foundation for the subgroups' activities, CDC conducted a systematic literature review that found more than 400 articles relevant to MTBI to be reviewed by subgroup members.

Definitions Subgroup

The Definitions Subgroup reviewed key literature from 1980 to 2001 to summarize clinical case definitions and diagnostic criteria for MTBI as a foundation for developing a conceptual definition of MTBI and for formulating operational definitions for important surveillance measures, such as incidence of medically-treated and non-treated cases and prevalence of disabilities.

Methods Subgroup

The Methods Subgroup reviewed key literature and data to identify potential surveillance databases and surveys to gather data about MTBI and its consequences. Subgroup members interviewed experts on databases and surveillance and evaluated systems using standard public health surveillance criteria (Teutsch 2000; CDC 2001); a summary of the evaluation criteria is found in Appendix B. They considered validity and reliability of data in making final recommendations. They also reviewed information about special populations, such as persons in school, special education classes, mental health institutions, and prisons.

Findings and Recommendations
of the CDC
Mild Traumatic Brain Injury Work Group

The subgroups met twice per month by teleconference from June 2001 to November 2001 to share information and to develop a plan for producing the Report to Congress. In late November 2001, the MTBI Work Group met with CDC staff in Atlanta to review findings and to formulate recommendations.

Definitions Subgroup Findings and Recommendations

The Definitions Subgroup found wide variation in the clinical case definitions and criteria used to identify MTBIs. As a foundation for developing operational definitions for MTBI, the subgroup developed conceptual definitions.

A **conceptual case definition** provides criteria to identify a case of MTBI for surveillance purposes based on selected clinical signs, symptoms, and neuroimaging. This definition is necessary as a reference standard for the evaluation of operational or working definitions of MTBI used by surveillance systems.

An **operational case definition** provides quantifiable criteria to consistently identify cases of MTBI for surveillance purposes when reviewing coded health care administrative databases, abstracting information from medical records, or analyzing data from surveys and personal interviews. Operational definitions should be designed to approximate the conceptual definition as closely as possible.

The Definitions Subgroup used the Traumatic Brain Injury (TBI) definition found in CDC's *Guidelines for Surveillance of Central Nervous System Injury* (Thurman, Sniezek, Johnson, Greenspan and Smith 1995) as the foundation for its definitions. However, that definition does not categorize injuries by severity and is not well suited for surveillance of less severe injuries that may not be treated in hospital settings.

The recommended definitions for MTBI were developed with the following premises in mind:

- TBI severity refers to the degree of brain trauma as it is assessed during the acute phase of injury. TBI severity assessment focuses on acute signs and symptoms indicating brain pathophysiology.

- TBI *severity* should be distinguished from TBI *outcome* (Dikmen and Levin 1993). Assessment of TBI outcome focuses on subacute or chronic signs and symptoms related to impairment and disability. TBI outcome is most relevant to measures of TBI prevalence.

- Major criteria for distinguishing levels of TBI severity are based primarily on the immediate effects of TBI on consciousness or cognition. In addition, focal signs and intracranial pathology (demonstrable on neuroimaging studies such as computed tomography) are considered.

- An incident case should meet either conceptual or operational definition criteria within the surveillance period.

- Some criteria for distinguishing grades of severity await further clinical study and more conclusive evidence.

Recommended Conceptual Definition of Incident Cases of MTBI

A case of MTBI is an occurrence of injury to the head resulting from blunt trauma or acceleration or deceleration forces with one or more of the following conditions attributable to the head injury during the surveillance period:

- Any period of observed or self-reported transient confusion, disorientation, or impaired consciousness;

- Any period of observed or self-reported dysfunction of memory (amnesia) around the time of injury;

- Observed signs of other neurological or neuropsychological dysfunction, such as—

  - Seizures acutely following head injury;
  - Among infants and very young children: irritability, lethargy, or vomiting following head injury;
  - Symptoms among older children and adults such as headache, dizziness, irritability, fatigue, or poor concentration, when identified soon after injury, can be used to support the diagnosis of mild TBI, but cannot be used to make the diagnosis in the absence of loss of consciousness or altered consciousness. Further research may provide additional guidance in this area.

- Any period of observed or self-reported loss of consciousness lasting 30 minutes or less.

More severe brain injuries were excluded from the definition of MTBI and include one or more of the following conditions attributable to the injury:

- Loss of consciousness lasting longer than 30 minutes;

- Post-traumatic amnesia lasting longer than 24 hours;

- Penetrating craniocerebral injury.

A wide range of severity and the possibility of further gradation exists within this definition. The Definitions Subgroup identified additional criteria that may further distinguish degrees of severity within the spectrum of mild TBI. Under this recommended definition, TBI cases with intracranial lesions demonstrated by neuroimaging studies (e.g., computed tomography) or with focal neurological deficits (e.g., hemiplegia) may still be considered mild if the criteria described previously are met. Some evidence, although inconsistent, indicates that such cases may have poorer outcomes (Williams, Levin and Eisenberg 1990; Dikmen and Temkin, unpublished data, 2001). To the extent allowed by data sources, TBI surveillance systems and epidemiological studies should obtain information about the presence of intracranial lesions, focal findings, and duration of unconsciousness in reported cases. Mild TBI cases with such abnormalities should be distinguished from cases without them in analyses of MTBI outcome. The value of such findings to predict outcome may be better defined by future research.

Recommended Operational Definitions of Incident Cases of MTBI

Three operational definitions are recommended for case ascertainment based on interviews and surveys; health care administrative data sets, such as hospital billing data; and clinical records, such as hospital medical record reviews or trauma registry data.

Interview/survey definition

A case of MTBI is recognized when a person surveyed or interviewed (or his or her proxy respondent) affirms the occurrence, within the period under surveillance, of a nonfatal injury to the head that is accompanied by:

- Criteria consistent with the recommended conceptual case definition (above);

- Loss of consciousness or altered consciousness;

- Loss of memory for events immediately before, during, or after the injury.

Surveys and interviews should ask whether health care professionals evaluated such injuries and, if so, what level of care was received. Where possible, analyses of data should distinguish between injuries receiving no medical care, non-hospital-based care, hospital ED care, inpatient hospital care of 24 hours or less, and inpatient hospital care of more than 24 hours. Occurrences of brain injury with inpatient hospital care of more than 24 hours may be classified as more severe (i.e., they do not meet the criteria for MTBI).

Administrative data definition for surveillance or research (ICD-9-CM)

A case of MTBI is recognized among persons treated in health care facilities who are assigned the following ICD-9-CM diagnostic codes (International Classification of Diseases 1989):

ICD-9-CM First Four Digits =	ICD-9-CM Fifth Digit =
800.0, 800.5, 801.0, 801.5, 803.0, 803.5, 804.0, 804.5, 850.0, 850.1, 850.5 or 850.9	0, 1, 2, 6, 9, or Missing
854.0	1, 2, 6, 9, or Missing
959.0*	1

*The current inclusion of code 959.01 (i.e., head injury, unspecified) in this definition is provisional. Although a recent clarification in the definition of this code is intended to exclude concussions, there is evidence that nosologists have been using it to code TBIs. Accordingly, this code may be removed from the recommended definition of mild TBI when there is evidence that in common practice nosologists no longer assign this code for TBI.

The codes in this table represent one possible approach for identifying MTBI using ICD-9-CM codes obtained from administrative records. Research is needed to determine the reliability and validity of these codes for defining MTBI. The full range of ICD-9-CM codes consistent with TBI of any severity is published in the CDC *Guidelines for Surveillance of Central Nervous System Injury* (Thurman, Sniezek, Johnson, Greenspan and Smith 1995).

Clinical records data definition

A case of MTBI is recognized when medical records document any one of the following:

- Criteria consistent with the recommended conceptual case definition (page 16);

- Glasgow Coma Scale (GCS) score between 13 and 15 assigned at the time of first medical evaluation at a health care facility (Teasdale and Jennett 1974; 1976);[2]

- Abbreviated Injury Severity (AIS) Scale score of 2 for the head region (Association for the Advancement of Automotive Medicine 1998).

Injuries accompanied by indicators of neurological deterioration during the course of acute care, such as cases in which subsequent GCS scores fall below 13 are excluded.

Recommended Conceptual Definition of Prevalent Cases of MTBI-Related Impairments, Functional Limitations, Disabilities, and Persistent Symptoms

A prevalent case of MTBI-related impairment, functional limitation, disability, or persistent symptoms is recognized among persons with a history of MTBI who are experiencing any degree of neurological or neuropsychological problem attributable to the MTBI.

Recommended Operational Definitions of Prevalent Cases of MTBI-Related Impairments, Functional Limitations, Disabilities, and Persistent Symptoms

Measuring the prevalence of MTBI-related impairments, functional limitations, disabilities, and persistent symptoms requires follow-up assessments after recovery from the acute phase of injury: for example, at three months, six months, and one year or longer after injury. Follow-up studies of representative samples of persons who

---

[2] The Glasgow Coma Scale is widely used in clinical practice to distinguish degrees of TBI severity. The routine recording of GCS scores by clinicians and the collection of GCS data by surveillance systems are strongly recommended.

Among children under 36 months, a pediatric coma scale can be used. Some scales are intended to approximate the GCS, with a score of 13 to 15 indicating a mild injury. See Hahn YS, Chyung C, Barthel MJ, et al. Head injuries in children under 36 months of age: demography and outcome. *Child's Nervous System* 1988;4:34–40. See also Simpson DA, Cockington RA, Hanieh A, et al. Head injuries in infants and young children: The value of the pediatric coma scale. Review of the literature and report on a study. *Child's Nervous System* 1991;7:183–90.

experience MTBI are needed to generate accurate estimates of prevalence. To date, most follow-up studies have focused on persons who have been hospitalized for TBI and whose injuries were more severe. Follow-up studies should include persons with less severe injuries and those who were not hospitalized for their TBI; the prevalence of TBI-related disability is assumed to be lower in this population.

No widely accepted, standard assessment tool currently exists to identify prevalent cases of MTBI-related impairment, functional limitation, disability, and persistent symptoms in population-based surveys. CDC proposes the following limited criteria for constructing an operational definition for such surveys, when respondents are persons with a history of MTBI or reliable proxy respondents:

- Current symptoms reported consequent to MTBI not present before injury or those made worse in severity or frequency by the MTBI:
  - Problems with memory
  - Problems with concentration
  - Problems with emotional control
  - Headaches
  - Fatigue
  - Irritability
  - Dizziness
  - Blurred vision
  - Seizures

- Current limitations in functional status reported consequent to MTBI:
  - Basic activities of daily living (e.g., personal care, ambulation, travel)
  - Major activities (e.g., work, school, homemaking)
  - Leisure and recreation
  - Social integration
  - Financial independence

Most of these symptoms and limitations are associated with many other conditions in addition to MTBI. This lack of specificity for MTBI places some limitations on the validity of studies of the prevalence of MTBI-related impairments, functional limitations, disabilities, and persistent symptoms. However, these limitations may be minimized by appropriate selection of comparison groups and cautious interpretation of findings, and by assessing pre- and post-injury symptom occurrence. If pre-existing symptoms cannot be "attributable" to the MTBI, these data should also be documented for further study and interpretation.

Methods Subgroup Findings and Recommendations

The Methods Subgroup reviewed a wide range of databases and surveys to identify those that would be most appropriate for measuring the incidence of MTBI; to determine the prevalence of MTBI-related impairments and disabilities; to determine underlying causes of MTBIs; and to identify population groups at risk regardless of age. Most of these databases and surveys were set up largely to provide information about other medical issues, but together, and with additional questions added, they can provide a more complete picture of MTBI. To obtain data on the incidence and prevalence of MTBI, established methods such as hospital emergency department- and hospital-based data collection and analysis should be the first priority. As resources and capacity will allow, the other methods provided in this report can serve as additional sources of good information. A summary of the subgroup's review and findings follows.

Detection and Surveillance of New Cases (Incidence) of Medically-Treated MTBI

In making recommendations for measuring the incidence of medically-treated MTBIs, the Methods Subgroup was primarily concerned with including data sources that are accessible, valid, and reliable. The recommendations focused largely on enhancing capabilities to conduct TBI surveillance in emergency departments (EDs), because many more MTBIs are diagnosed and treated in EDs than in hospital inpatient settings and because such ED data systems already exist in some states and at the national level. However, the subgroup also recognized the need to improve surveillance of hospitalized cases of MTBI. Specific recommendations include:

Priority Recommendations to Obtain Data on the Incidence and Prevalence of MTBI

- Increase the number of states conducting ED-based TBI surveillance using the South Carolina Department of Health (SC DOH) TBI Surveillance Program as a model.

- Routinely analyze data from CDC's National Hospital Ambulatory Medical Care Survey (NHAMCS) and National Ambulatory Medical Care Survey (NAMCS) to estimate incidence of, study external causes related to, and identify trends in MTBIs treated in, outpatient settings.

- Increase the number of states conducting MTBI surveillance using hospital discharge data.

- Consider using large, national hospital discharge databases, such as the Nation-wide Inpatient Sample database [conducted by the Agency for Health Care Research and Quality (AHRQ)/Healthcare Cost and Utilization Project (HCUP)] that have not been used previously for injury surveillance.

- Explore using data from the National Electronic Injury Surveillance System (NEISS) to assess the incidence and external causes of MTBI in the United States among persons treated in EDs.

Additional Recommendations

- Routinely analyze data collected by CDC's National Health Interview Survey (NHIS) to estimate the incidence of MTBI among persons who receive medical care outside of hospitals and hospital EDs.

- Analyze data from the National Collegiate Athletic Association Injury Surveillance System (NCAAISS) to assess the incidence of MTBI among participants in selected college sports.

- Apply the recommended operational definition of MTBI to enhance the capability of current CDC-funded state TBI Surveillance Systems and other national and state hospital discharge databases to detect and monitor MTBI incidence.

- Routinely analyze data from the National Hospital Discharge Survey (NHDS) to assess hospitalization patterns due to MTBI.

- Collaborate with the Defense and Veterans Head Injury Program to use use their database and the Defense and Medical Surveillance System databases to determine the occurrence of MTBI in these systems.

Detection and Surveillance of New Cases (Incidence) of MTBI Not Receiving Medical Care

Measuring the incidence of MTBIs that are not treated medically is difficult because the injuries are not documented in any routinely-collected health information system. To the extent possible, the Methods Subgroup considered ways to add modules to existing surveys or studies. Specific recommendations include the following:

- Explore adding MTBI-related questions to large, existing state-based surveys, such as those conducted through CDC's Behavioral Risk Factor Surveillance System (BRFSS) and Youth Risk Behavior Surveillance System (YRBSS).

- Explore adding a module to CDC's National Health Interview Survey (NHIS) to study the incidence, external causes, and the consequences of MTBI among persons in the community, including those who did not receive medical care.

- For a sample of individuals self-reporting the receipt of medical care as a result of MTBI (identified via NHIS-DS and BRFSS), special follow-up studies with health care providers will be considered to determine the accuracy of self-reporting.

Identifying and Assessing Prevalent Cases of MTBI-Related Impairment, Functional Limitation, Disability, and Persistent Symptoms

Identifying individuals disabled by the effects of a MTBI presents a challenge not only because they are not routinely documented in current health information systems, but also because many of the impairments, functional limitations, disabilities, and persistent symptoms experienced by persons with MTBI, may result from other conditions. Most existing health information systems and surveys are inadequate for this type of surveillance. Thus, documenting who and how many people are disabled by MTBI-related problems will be more costly than the surveillance and study of acute, medically-treated cases. With these considerations in mind, the Methods Subgroup recommended the following:

- Explore adding MTBI-related questions to existing surveys, such as the National Health Interview Survey–Disability Supplement (NHIS-DS), to determine the prevalence of individuals with MTBI-related functional and cognitive impairments or disabilities.

- Determine the feasibility of adding MTBI disability questions to state-based surveillance systems or surveys, such as BRFSS.

- For a sample of individuals self-reporting the receipt of medical care as a result of MTBI (identified via NHIS-DS and BRFSS), special follow-up studies with health care providers should be considered to determine the accuracy of self-reporting.

- Consider determining the occurrence of MTBI-related disabilities and impairments among children by adding questions to large, longitudinal studies such as the 30-year follow-up National Children's Study (http://nationalchildrensstudy.gov).

- Collaborate with the Defense and Veterans Head Injury Program to use their database and the Defense and Medical Surveillance System databases to determine the occurrence of MTBI-related disabilities.

- Use existing TBI surveillance systems and registries to develop prospective follow-up studies to determine what percentage of persons with MTBI become disabled or experience persistent symptoms, to identify which cases receive appropriate services, and to link brain-injured persons with appropriate rehabilitation support and other services.

Establishing the Natural History of MTBI-Related Disabilities and Impairments

Health care providers need a better understanding of the progression of acute injury into long-term disability to identify brain-injured persons at greatest risk for lasting problems and to determine when to intervene to ensure the best possible outcomes. This knowledge will be gained through studying patients with MTBI over time. To this end, the Methods Subgroup focused on using existing or proposed databases and studies capable of tracking MTBI cases from occurrence to two or more years after injury. Specific recommendations include the following:

- Collaborate with the Defense and Veterans Head Injury Program to use their database to determine the natural history of MTBIs experienced by military personnel and to identify pre-existing, acute, and chronic factors that predict the likelihood of disabilities, impairments, and persistent symptoms.

- Explore adding MTBI-related questions to longitudinal studies, such as the National Children's Study to track the evolution of symptoms and disabilities associated with MTBI.

- Support the development of state-based TBI registries with the ability to track acute MTBI cases longitudinally.

- Develop methods to determine the effects of pre-injury conditions, such as learning disabilities and psychiatric problems, and post-injury conditions and circumstances, such as depression, substance abuse, and compensation.

The relationship of symptoms and their resolution to the presence of biological markers that may be developed in the future, is an important research question that also needs to be addressed.

Documenting the Prevalence of Individuals with MTBI-Related Disabilities in Special Populations

Documenting the prevalence of individuals impaired by MTBIs in special populations— such as those in school programs, mental health institutions, and prisons—is difficult for several reasons. First, there is a lack of standardized definitions for special populations. Second, no health data systems exist for these populations specifically. Finally, in many cases, no data of any kind exist about MTBI among these groups. For these reasons, the Methods Subgroup determined that information about special populations is not of sufficient quantity or quality to make recommendations at this time. Given the current knowledge in these areas, stakeholders should coordinate activities to promote research and to standardize data collection instruments and methods.

Conclusion

Evidence indicates that MTBI is a public health problem, the magnitude and impact of which are underestimated by current surveillance systems. Much research is needed to determine the full magnitude of MTBI, to identify preventable and modifiable risk factors, and to develop and test strategies to reduce MTBIs and to improve outcomes for those who sustain these injuries. Such research will inform the development of more effective primary prevention strategies and policies to address the service and rehabilitation needs of persons with MTBI. The recommendations in this report can help shape that research.

Already, the definitions of MTBI recommended in this report have received support from the public health community. The World Health Organization's Task Force on Mild Traumatic Brain Injury reviewed the definitions, and, at the time this report was prepared, recommended that these definitions be used worldwide for surveillance purposes. This recommendation is an important first step in establishing acceptance of uniform definitions of MTBI.

References

Adelson PD, Kochanek PM. Head injury in children. J Child Neurol 1998;13:2–15.

Alexander MP. Mild traumatic brain injury: pathophysiology, natural history, and clinical management. Neurology 1995;45:1253–60.

Alves W, Macciocchi SN, Barth JT. Postconcussive symptoms after uncomplicated mild head injury. J Head Trauma Rehabil 1993;8(3)48–59.

American Congress of Rehabilitation Medicine. Definition of mild traumatic brain injury. J Head Trauma Rehabil 1993;8:86–8.

Association for the Advancement of Automotive Medicine. The Abbreviated Injury Scale, 1990 Revision. Barrington (IL): (UpDate); 1998.

Barsky AJ, Borus JF. Functional somatic syndromes. Ann Intern Med 1999;130:910–21.

Barth JT, Macciocchi SN, Giordani B, Rimel R, Jane JA, Boll TJ. Neuropsychological sequelae of minor head injury. Neurosurgery 1983;13:529–33.

Beattie TF. Minor head injury. Arch Dis Child 1997;77:82–5.

Bernstein DM. Recovery from mild head injury. Brain Inj 1999;13:151–72.

Bigler ED, Snyder JL. Neuropsychological outcome and quantitative neuroimaging in mild head injury. Arch Clin Neuropsychol 1995;10:159–74.

Binder LM, Rohling ML, Larrabee GJ. A review of mild head trauma. Part I: Meta-analytic review of neuropsychological studies. J Clin Exp Neuropsychol 1997;3:421–31.

Bohnen N, Twijnstra A, Jolles J. Post-traumatic and emotional symptoms in different subgroups of patients with mild head injury. Brain Inj 1992;6:481–7.

CDC. Traumatic brain injury in the United States: A Report to Congress. Atlanta (GA): Centers for Disease Control and Prevention, National Center for Injury Prevention and Control; 1999.

CDC. Updated guidelines for evaluating public health surveillance systems. Recommendations from the guidelines working group. MMWR 2001;50(RR13):1–35.

Culotta VP, Sementilli ME, Gerold K, Watts CC. Clinicopathological heterogeneity in the classification of mild head injury. Neurosurgery 1996;38:245–50.

Deb S, Lyons I, Koutzoukis C. Neuropsychiatric sequelae one year after a minor head injury. J Neurol Neurosurg Psychiatry 1998;65:899–902.

De Kruijk JR, Twijnstra A, Leffers P. Diagnostic criteria and differential diagnosis of mild traumatic brain injury. Brain Inj 2001;15:99–106.

Dikmen SS, Levin HS. Methodological issues in the study of mild head injury. J Head Trauma Rehabil 1993;8(3):30–7.

Guerrero JL, Thurman DJ, Sniezek JE. Emergency department visits associated with traumatic brain injury: United States, 1995–1996. Brain Inj 2000;14:181–6.

Guthkelch AN. Posttraumatic amnesia, postconcussional symptoms and accident neurosis. Eur Neurol 1980;19:91–102.

Hahn YS, Chyung C, Barthel MJ, Bailes J, Flannery AM, McLone DG. Head injuries in children under 36 months of age: demography and outcome. Child's Nerv Syst 1988; 4:34–40.

Ingebrigtsen T, Romner B, Marup-Jensen S, Dons M, Lundqvist C, Bellner J, et al. The clinical value of serum S-100 protein measurements in minor head injury: a Scandinavian multicentre study. Brain Inj 2000;14(12):1047–55.

International Classification of Diseases, Ninth Revision, Clinical Modification, 3rd ed. (ICD-9-CM). Washington (DC): Department of Health and Human Services; 1989.

Iverson GL, McCracken LM. 'Postconcussive' symptoms in persons with chronic pain. Brain Inj 1997;11:783–90.

Jennett B. Epidemiology of head injury. J Neurol Neurosurg Psychiatry 1996;60:362–9.

Kibby MY, Long CJ. Minor head injury: attempts at clarifying the confusion. Brain Inj 1996;10(3):159–86. Review.

Kraus JF, Fife D, Conroy C. Pediatric brain injuries: the nature, clinical course, and early outcomes in a defined United States' population. Pediatrics 1987;79:501–7.

Kraus JF, McArthur DL, Silberman TA. Epidemiology of Mild Brain Injury. Semin Neurol 1994;14:1–7.

Kurtzke JF, Jurland LT. The Epidemiology of neurologic disease. In: Joynt RJ, editor. Clin Neurol, Rev. Philadelphia: JB Lippincott; 1993.

Kushner D. Mild traumatic brain injury: toward understanding manifestations and treatment. Arch Intern Medicine 1998;158(15):1617–24.

Macciocchi SN, Barth JT, Littlefield LM. Outcome after mild head injury. Clin Sports Med 1998;17(1):27–36.

Max W, MacKenzie EJ, Rice DP. Head injuries: costs and consequences. J Head Trauma Rehabil 1991;6(2):76–91.

Rimel RW, Giordani B, Barth JT, Boll TJ, Jane JA. Disability caused by minor head injury. Neurosurgery 1981;9:221–8.

Rimel RW, Giordani B, Barth JT, Jane JA. Moderate head injury: completing the clinical spectrum of brain trauma. Neurosurgery 1982;11:344–51.

Ruff R, Jurica P. In search of a unified definition for mild traumatic brain injury. Brain Inj 1999;3(12):943–52.

Russell WR. The traumatic amnesias. London: Oxford University Press; 1971.

Rutherford WH. Postconcussion symptoms: relationship to acute neurological indices, individual differences, and circumstances of injury. In: Levin HS, Eisenberg HM, Benton AL, editors. Mild Head Injury. New York: Oxford University Press; 1989. p. 217–28.

Rutherford WH, Merrett JD, McDonald JR. Symptoms at one year following concussion from minor head injuries. Injury 1978;10:225–30.

Simpson DA, Cockington RA, Hanieh A, Raftos J, Reilly PL. Head injuries in infants and young children: the value of the pediatric coma scale. Review of the literature and report on a study. Child's Nerv Syst 1991;7:183–90.

Sosin DM, Sniezek JE, Thurman DJ. Incidence of mild and moderate brain injury in the United States, 1991. Brain Inj 1996;10:47–54.

Steadman JH, Graham JG. Head injuries: an analysis and follow-up study. Proc R Soc Med 1970;63:23–8.

Swift TL, Wilson SL. Misconceptions about brain injury among the general public and non-expert health professionals: an exploratory study. Brain Inj 2001;15:149–65.

Teasdale G, Jennett B. Assessment of coma and impaired consciousness: a practical scale. Lancet 1974;2:81–4.

Teasdale G, Jennett B. Assessment and prognosis of coma after head injury. Acta Neurochir (Wien) 1976;34:45–55.

Tellier A, Della Malva LC, Cwinn A, Grahovac S, Morrish W, Brennan-Barnes M. Mild head injury: a misnomer. Brain Inj 1999;13:463–75.

Teutsch SM. Considerations in planning a surveillance system. In: Teutsch SM, Churchill RE, editors. Principles and Practice of Public Health Surveillance. 2nd edition. New York: Oxford University Press; 2000. p. 17–29.

Thurman DJ, Branche CM, Sniezek JE. The epidemiology of sports-related traumatic brain injuries in the United States: recent developments. J Head Trauma Rehabil 1998; 13(2):1–8.

Thurman D, Guerrero J. Trends in hospitalization associated with traumatic brain injury. JAMA 1999;282:954–7.

Thurman DJ, Sniezek JE, Johnson D, Greenspan A, Smith SM. Guidelines for Surveillance of Central Nervous System Injury. Atlanta (GA): Centers for Disease Control and Prevention; 1995.

Thurman DJ. The epidemiology and economics of head trauma. In: Miller L, Hayes R, editors. Head Trauma: Basic, Preclinical, and Clinical Directions. New York: John Wiley and Sons; 2001.

Wessely S, Nimnuan C, Sharpe M. Functional somatic syndromes: one or many? Lancet 1999;354:936–9.

Williams DH, Levin HS, Eisenberg HM. Mild health injury classification. Neurosurgery 1990;217(3):442–8.

Appendix A:
CDC Mild Traumatic Brain Injury
Work Group

Senior Editor

Victor G. Coronado, M.D., M.P.H.
Medical Epidemiologist
Division of Injury and Disability Outcomes and Programs
National Center for Injury Prevention and Control
Centers for Disease Control and Prevention
Atlanta, Georgia

Editor

Bruce Jones, M.D., M.P.H.
Acting Team Leader
Disability and Rehabilitation Team
Division of Injury and Disability Outcomes and Programs
National Center for Injury Prevention and Control
Centers for Disease Control and Prevention
Atlanta, Georgia

Executive Secretary

Victor G. Coronado, M.D., M.P.H.
Medical Epidemiologist
Division of Injury and Disability Outcomes and Programs
National Center for Injury Prevention and Control
Centers for Disease Control and Prevention
Atlanta, Georgia

Definitions Subgroup

Jeffrey J. Bazarian, M.D.
Assistant Professor
University of Rochester Medical Center
Department of Emergency Medicine
Rochester, New York

Kathleen R. Bell, M.D.
Associate Professor
Department of Rehabilitation Medicine
University of Washington Medical Center
Seattle, Washington

Jörgen Borg, M.D.
Associate Professor, Neurology, Karolinska Institutet
Head, Department of Rehabilitation Medicine
Stockholm, Sweden

Sureyya Dikmen, Ph.D.
Professor, Department of Rehabilitation Medicine
Neurological Surgery and Psychiatry and Behavioral Sciences
University of Washington
Seattle, Washington

Jess F. Kraus, Ph.D., M.P.H.
Director, Southern California Injury Prevention Research Center
UCLA School of Public Health
Los Angeles, California

Charles J. Long, Ph.D.
Chair, Director, MS Graduate Psychology Program
Psychology Department
The University of Memphis
Memphis, Tennessee

David Thurman, M.D.
Medical Epidemiologist
National Center for Chronic Disease Prevention and Health Promotion
Centers for Disease Control and Prevention
Atlanta, Georgia

Methods Subgroup

Robert C. Cantu, M.D.
Medical Director
National Center for Catastrophic Sports Injury Research
University of North Carolina
Chief, Neurosurgery Service
Emerson Hospital
Concord, Massachusetts

J. David Cassidy, Ph.D.
Associate Professor, Epidemiology and Medicine
Alberta Centre for Injury Control and Research
Department of Public Health Sciences
Faculty, Medicine and Dentistry
University of Alberta
Edmonton, Alberta, Canada

John D. Corrigan, Ph.D.
Professor, Department of Physical Medicine and Rehabilitation
The Ohio State University
Columbus, Ohio

Virginia M. Lesser, Dr.P.H., M.S.
Assistant Professor, Statistics
Director, Survey Research Center
Oregon State University
Corvallis, Oregon

Gregory O'Shanick, M.D.
Co-Chair, U.S. Mild Traumatic Brain Injury (MTBI)
Guideline Development Work Group
National Medical Director, Brain Injury Association of America
Medical Director, Center for Neuro-Rehabilitation Services
Midlothian, Virginia

Peter Patrick, Ph.D.
Associate Professor, Clinical Pediatrics
School of Medicine, University of Virginia
Director, Pediatric Psychology/Neuropsychology
Children's Medical Center
Kluge Children's Rehabilitation Center
Charlottesville, Virginia

Karen Schwab, Ph.D.
Assistant Director for Statistics
Defense and Veterans Head Injury Program
Department of Neurology
Walter Reed Army Medical Center
Gaithersburg, Maryland

Anbesaw W. Selassie, Dr.P.H.
Chair, Department of Biometry and Epidemiology
Medical University of South Carolina
Charleston, South Carolina

Nancy Temkin, Ph.D.
Associate Professor, Neurological Surgery and Biostatistics
Department of Neurological Surgery
University of Washington
Seattle, Washington

Barbara Weissman, M.D.
Associate Professor Pediatrics (Neurology)
Emory University School of Medicine
Medical Director, Rehabilitation Services
Children's Healthcare of Atlanta at Egleston
Medical Director, Day RehabilitationProgram
Children's Healthcare of Atlanta
Atlanta, Georgia

Appendix B:
Criteria Used to Evaluate Proposed, Ongoing Surveillance Systems to Identify Persons with Mild Traumatic Brain Injury in the United States

The following criteria are summarized from CDC guidelines for evaluating public health surveillance systems (CDC 2001).

Simplicity. Structure and ease of operating the surveillance system. Is the operational case definition easy to apply? Are cases easily ascertained? How much time and how many resources are or will be required to maintain the system?

Flexibility. System's ability to adapt as information needs or operating conditions change, given limited availability of personnel and/or funds.

Data Quality. Completeness and accuracy of the data collected. What is the proportion of unknown and missing responses?

Acceptability. Willingness of the survey population to participate in the surveillance system. What are the participation rates? What are the interview completion rates and refusal rates?

Sensitivity. System's ability to detect true cases of MTBI. What is the proportion of cases detected? How well can the system track changes and trends over time?

Predictive Value Positive. Proportion of reported cases that actually experienced the health event or have the health condition under surveillance.

Representativeness. Accuracy of a system to describe the occurrence of a health event or condition under surveillance over time and its distribution in the population by place and person.

Timeliness. Speed between steps in public health surveillance from the occurrence of the event to feedback to clinicians, investigators, legislators, and the public.

Stability. System's ability to collect, manage, and report data properly without failure.

Appendix C:
Descriptions of Recommended
Mild Traumatic Brain Injury Databases

South Carolina Department of Health (SC DOH)
TBI Surveillance System

Characteristics: Statewide surveillance system conducted by the SC DOH with CDC funds since 1995 to characterize the epidemiology of TBI in this state. Targets all state residents, regardless of age, who receive health care in hospitals and in self-standing or hospital-based EDs. Data are abstracted from coded hospital discharge and ED administrative databases. Medical records are reviewed for a sample. Data are unduplicated (thus, it is a true patient-level). Coded mortality data is also collected. It requires $300,000 to $370,000 a year ($150,000 to $200,000 for ED data and $150,000 to $170,000 for hospital and vital statistics data).

Strengths: Population-based. State representative. Targets all ages. Timely. Economical. Includes ED-based data. Reports true, unduplicated cases. Uses International Classification of Diseases, Ninth Revision, Clinical Modification (ICD-9-CM) rubrics to code medical diagnoses.

Limitations: If implemented in other states, a law requiring all self-standing and hospital-based EDs to report in standard format may be necessary.

Recommendations: Use as model to be implemented in selected states. Allows the yearly study of incidence, trends, demographics, external causes, and selected risk factors in the population. Potential use for follow-up studies to improve understanding of the natural history of MTBI.

National Electronic Injury Surveillance System (NEISS)

Characteristics: Nationally-representative, probability sample surveillance system of all U.S. hospitals with EDs conducted by the U.S. Consumer Product Safety Commission since 1972 and expanded through collaboration with CDC in July 2000. Targets all persons regardless of age who receive health care in 100 representative hospital-based EDs. NEISS collects data for over 500,000 cases per year, visiting selected EDs. Trained NEISS staff abstract data daily from eligible records. Subsequent telephone or on-site follow-back interviews yield clues about the causes of injury. Only first-time-visit data are reported. Routine analysis of NEISS data costs $100,000 to $150,000 per year.

Strengths: Nationally representative. Large population under study may allow better estimates. Targets all ages. Timely. Economical. Has a follow-back system. Identifies unduplicated cases. Provides patient-level data.

Limitations: Coding accuracy varies by variable from 27 percent (for adverse effects) to 92 percent (for transportation-related cases). Has its own special coding system different from that of the International Classification of Diseases, Ninth Revision, Clinical Modification (ICD-9-CM).

Recommendations: Analyze routinely to study incidence, external causes, occupation and type of industry, and risk factors. Potential uses for follow-up or follow-back studies to assess the natural history of MTBI.

National Hospital Ambulatory Medical Care Survey (NHAMCS) – Emergency Department and Outpatient Department Modules

Characteristics: Nationally-representative, four-stage probability sample survey of visits to hospital EDs and outpatient departments (ODs) of non-federal, short-stay general hospitals in the United States. Conducted by CDC's National Center for Health Statistics since 1992. Targets all persons regardless of age who receive health care in hospital-based EDs and ODs. Hospital staff collects health care information for all visits to EDs and ODs during a randomly assigned four week reporting period. Sample data are weighted to produce annual, nationally-representative estimates. Routine analysis of NHAMCS data costs $100,000 to $150,000 per year. Adding more variables to obtain two more diagnostic codes costs $100,000 per year.

Strengths: Nationally representative. Targets all ages. Timely. Economical. Uses International Classification of Diseases, Ninth Revision, Clinical Modification (ICD-9-CM) rubrics to code medical diagnoses.

Limitations: Only three diagnostic codes are collected; thus, MTBI cases may be missed (estimated missing cases range from 25 to 30 percent). Production of more precise estimates requires aggregating data from at least two survey years.

Recommendations: Analyze routinely (at intervals of at least two years) to study incidence, trends, demographics, external causes of injury, service use, hospital characteristics, expected source of payment, chief complaint and diagnosis, medications, type of provider, and disposition of MTBI-related visits to EDs and ODs. Additional funds will be necessary to collect at least five diagnostic codes; this will allow detection of 90 to 95 percent of all MTBIs.

National Ambulatory Medical Care Survey (NAMCS)

Characteristics: Nationally-representative, multistage probability sample survey of visits to the offices of non-federally employed physicians (excluding those in anesthesiology, radiology, and pathology), including visits to non-hospital-based clinics and health maintenance organizations. Conducted by CDC's National Center for Health Statistics since 1973. Targets all persons regardless of age who receive health care from selected office-based physicians. Health data for a systematic random sample of office visits occurring during a randomly assigned one-week reporting period are abstracted by sampled physicians (1,088 in 1999). Routine analysis of the NAMCS costs $100,000 to $150,000 yearly.

Strengths: Nationally representative. Targets persons of all ages. Economical. Uses International Classification of Diseases, Ninth Revision, Clinical Modification (ICD-9-CM) rubrics to code medical diagnoses.

Limitations: Only three diagnostic codes are collected; thus, MTBI cases may be missed. Excludes specialties of radiology, anesthesiology, and pathology. Precise estimates require aggregating data from at least two consecutive years.

Recommendations: Analyze routinely (at intervals of at least two years) to study incidence, trends, demographics, reasons for visits, place of injury, use of preventive services (including violence and injury prevention), medications, and disposition of MTBI-related visits.

National Health Interview Survey (NHIS)

Characteristics: Population-based, nationally-representative, face-to-face area probability sample survey conducted by CDC's National Center for Health Statistics since 1957. Used to assess public health issues among the civilian, non-institutionalized U.S. population. Respondents are household residents ages 18 years and older. Data is obtained for all members of the family residing in the household; respondents are the proxies for younger persons living in the household. Topical data (e.g., disability) are collected. In 1997, data from 40,000 households were collected; 103,5000 persons responded to the interview. The Injury Section of the Core NHIS Instrument identifies injuries requiring medical attention occurring in the three months preceding the interview among respondents or family members residing in the household at the time of the interview. Causes and consequences of each injury episode are also collected. Routine analysis of the NHIS data costs $100,000 to $150,000 per year.

Strengths: Population based. Nationally representative. Targets all ages. Economical. Potential use for follow-up; costs for this aspect were not estimated at this time. Uses International Classification of Diseases, Ninth Revision, Clinical Modification (ICD-9-CM) rubrics to code medical diagnoses.

Limitations: Current care-of-injury eligibility criteria exclude people who did not receive health care or advice. Current time-of-injury eligibility criteria (i.e., injuries requiring medical attention occurring in the three months preceding the interview) limit study of the natural history and sample size. Any proposed follow-up study requires funding and up to two to three years for implementation.

Recommendations: Analyze routinely to study incidence, trends, and demographics. Data from the Disability Supplement can also be analyzed routinely. Findings can also be compared with methods of contemporaneous surveillance of health events and can serve as a validation system. Propose modifying current care-of-injury eligibility criteria to allow for identification and interview of persons who had a MTBI but did not receive medical care or advice. Extend current time-of-injury eligibility criteria to generate a larger sample. Follow-up studies can be proposed and implemented, provided that questions regarding natural history and associated disability are included in the instrument.

National Collegiate Athletic Association Injury Surveillance System (NCAAISS)

Characteristics: Population-based, nationally-representative sports-related injury surveillance system that has collected data from a representative sample of colleges that are members of the National Collegiate Athletic Association (NCAA) since 1982 (450 of 977 in 2000). Final selection of participant colleges is random and includes at least 10 percent of each NCAA division. Data are used to reduce injury through changes in rules, protective equipment, and coaching techniques. Targets college students practicing spring football; wrestling; baseball; ice and field hockey; women's volleyball and softball; and men's and women's soccer, basketball, gymnastics, and Lacrosse. Data on at least one sport are collected in a standardized questionnaire by certified and student athletic trainers from the first official day of pre-season practice to the final tournament contest.

Strengths: Population based. NCAA representative. Conducted at no cost to CDC. Can produce regional and state-level estimates. Potential use for follow-up studies.

Limitations: Excludes all non-NCAA colleges. Does not include some contact sports (e.g., karate). Data are not validated.

Recommendations: Analyze routinely to assess the incidence of MTBI in selected college sports. Follow-up/follow-back studies can be added; these enhancements will allow clinicians and investigators to characterize natural history, adverse outcomes, and associated disability.

CDC Traumatic Brain Injury Surveillance System

Characteristics: Statewide, representative surveillance system conducted in selected states receiving CDC funding since 1996. This system is the only ongoing, population-based TBI surveillance system in the United States. It has two aspects: core surveillance, which relies on International Classification of Diseases, Version 9, Clinical Modification codes found in hospital discharge and vital statistics data; and extended surveillance, which relies on abstraction of relevant health information via medical record review. Targets hospitalized persons regardless of age. During the funding cycle that ended in 2000, 15 states received funds to conduct the core aspect; 14 of these also conducted the expanded aspect. In the cycle that began in late 2000, only 12 states were funded to conduct core TBI surveillance; of these, six were funded to conduct expanded surveillance. This system requires $140,000 to $180,000 per state per year ($80,000 to $100,000 to conduct the core aspect and $60,000 to $80,000 to conduct the expanded surveillance aspect).

Strengths: Representative at the state level. Economical. Targets persons of all ages. Uses International Classification of Diseases, Ninth Revision, Clinical Modification (ICD-9-CM) rubrics to code medical diagnoses. Potential use for follow-up studies.

Limitations: Not timely. Current TBI definition is not suitable for detecting cases of MTBI. Does not include ED data.

Recommendations: Analyze routinely to assess incidence, external causes, and risk factors of MTBI among persons who are hospitalized. Apply the recommended definitions for MTBI to enhance the system's ability to detect and monitor MTBI in the United States. Increase the number of states conducting TBI surveillance.

National Hospital Discharge Survey (NHDS)

Characteristics: Nationally-representative, three-stage stratified sample survey of inpatient records acquired from a representative probability sample of about 500 non-federal, short-stay hospitals (average length of stay of 30 days or shorter) having six or more beds in the United States. Conducted by CDC's National Center for Health Statistics (NCHS) since 1965. The NHDS is designed to provide information about characteristics of inpatients (regardless of age) hospitalized and discharged from the hospitals in the survey. Medical and administrative data—including date of birth, sex, race, ethnicity, marital status, ZIP codes, dates of admission and discharge, discharge status, expected source of payment, procedures, diagnoses, size of hospital, and hospital ownership—for approximately 300,000 hospital discharges are obtained from two sources. The first source uses data that is manually-abstracted and transcribed by hospital and U.S. Bureau of the Census staff from a manually-selected sample of hospital discharge records. Completed forms are coded, computerized, and edited by NCHS. The second source uses a systematic sample of electronic hospital discharge files containing medical record data selected from electronic files purchased from public and private organizations authorized by the states. Approximately 10 percent of the abstracts are independently recoded with an overall error of 0.6 percent for medical coding and 0.3 percent for administrative coding. Approximately 40 percent of respondent hospitals provided data through the automated system. Sample data are weighted to produce annual, nationally-representative estimates. Routine analysis of NHDS data costs $100,000 to $150,000 per year.

Strengths: Nationally representative. Targets all ages. Excellent quality. Timely. Economical. Uses International Classification of Diseases, Ninth Revision, Clinical Modification (ICD-9-CM) rubrics to code medical diagnoses.

Limitations: Does not include ED data. Cannot distinguish first admissions from readmissions in some states; thus, allowing for discharge rates, not injury rates. Measures discharges and not individual patients (potential duplicates).

Recommendations: Analyze routinely to study incidence, trends, demographics, external causes of injury, service use, hospital characteristics, expected source of payment, chief complaint and diagnosis, medications, type of provider, and disposition of MTBI-related hospitalizations in non-federal, short-stay hospitals in the United States.

Nationwide Inpatient Sample (NIS)

Characteristics: Nationally-representative, multi-state health data system based on all hospital discharges from a stratified probability sample of non-federal, short-stay hospitals (994 in 28 participant states in 2000). Sponsored by the Agency for Healthcare Research and Quality since 1988. Designed to approximate a 20 percent sample of all non-federal, short-term, general and other specialty hospitals in the United States. The NIS 2000 is a sample of hospitals that comprise about 80 percent of all hospital discharges in the United States. States voluntarily report allowable electronic, coded discharge data from all persons hospitalized regardless of age. Analysis of NIS data costs $100,000 to $150,000 annually.

Strengths: Representative at the participant state and national levels. Economical. Targets persons of all ages. Contains data on discharge disposition, procedures, service use, length of hospitalization, source of payment, and costs among hospitalized persons with MTBI at the national level. Contains 7 million records (in contrast, the National Hospital Discharge Survey (NHDS) contains 300,000). Uses International Classification of Diseases, Ninth Revision, Clinical Modification (ICD-9-CM) rubrics to code medical diagnoses.

Limitations: Does not include ED data. Reporting is not uniform: small hospitals are underrepresented in some states; hospitals in some states report only a subset of their discharges. Cannot distinguish first admissions from readmissions in some states; thus, allowing for discharge rates, not injury rates. Measures discharges and not individual patients (potential duplicates).

Recommendations: Analyze routinely to study the incidence of MTBI-related hospitalization and discharge in non-federal, short-stay hospitals in the United States.

Behavioral Risk Factor Surveillance System (BRFSS) and the South Carolina Department of Health Interagency Office of Disability and Health Disability Surveillance (SC DOH IODH-DS)

Characteristics: CDC-sponsored, population-based, random digit dialing telephone surveillance system that collects topical data about varying health issues, including disability, among persons in the community. Includes persons who did not seek medical care. SC DOH IODH-DS has used BRFSS since the early 1990s, including a question about the likely cause of any disability in the "Quality of Life and Care Giving" module. BRFSS targets primarily people ages 18 years and older; however, some states collect infor-mation about children from parents or legal guardians. Costs vary with the number of questions added to the data collection instrument. Adding questions and administering them to the target population costs $35,000 to $50,000 per question. Routine data analy-sis costs $50,000 to $70,000 per year.

Strengths: Population based. Representative at the state level; nationally representative if questions are administered by all participating states. Relatively economical. Allows identification of cases of persons with MTBI who did not receive health care. Potential use for follow-up studies among both adults and children.

Limitations: Nationally representative only if questions are administered by all states. Question about the likely cause of any disability in the "Quality of Life and Care Giving" module has low completion rates; thus, it needs to be re-written and tested. Does not cover population of persons in households without phones.

Recommendations: Injury-related questions or module can be added to the data collection instrument and used to study MTBI incidence in the community, especially among those who did not receive health care (requires pre-testing of proposed questions before administering them in states). Follow-up studies can also be proposed.

National Children's Study (NCS)

Characteristics: Planned, population-based, nationally-representative, longitudinal cohort study of 100,000 children (from birth to adulthood) to measure exposure of risks for asthma, unintentional injuries, cancer, and developmental disorders; to assess outcomes of such health and safety problems; and to identify factors for improving children's health and well being. Children will be recruited, measured, and followed-up in geographically-distributed centers using sampling techniques. Special populations will be oversampled. The National Institute of Child Health and Human Development (part of the National Institutes of Health), the Environmental Protection Agency (EPA), and CDC are leading a consortium of federal and non-federal partners. It includes children, their families, and their environment, physical, chemical, biological, and psychosocial influences. Biomarkers and exposure measurements will be collected and evaluated. Methodological development and pilot studies began in FY 2001 and will run through FY 2003; the study should begin in 2004 and is expected to end by 2035.

Strengths: Population based. Nationally representative. Targets children and their families. Hypothesis driven. Longitudinal design allows for determining causality and natural history. Biomarkers will be used. Special populations will be oversampled. Study design allows pilot tests to recommend standard tests or measures. CDC will incur no costs.

Limitations: Not a tested system. Excludes intentional injuries. Preliminary finding and results will not be available until 2010.

Recommendations: CDC should ensure the inclusion of a follow-up component to study the incidence and the natural history of MTBI among children in the United States. A pilot study could develop an injury severity scale to measure the long-term cognitive outcomes for MTBI, especially the cumulative effects of repetitive injuries (e.g., multiple minor concussions). In addition, a scale could distinguish between acute and chronic injuries; however, this distinction does not relate to outcome.

Defense and Veterans Head Injury Program (DVHIP)

Characteristics: Military and VA beneficiary TBI registry, based on patient information from seven lead sites and 20 network sites in the DVHIP. Conducted by the Department of Defense (DoD) and the Department of Veterans Affairs (VA) sites of the DVHIP since 1992. Data collected include those from standardized evaluation batteries, randomized trials, and data from the Defense National Databases. Components considered to study MTBI are primarily found among military patients included in the TBI registry and the DoD and VA national discharge databases for incidence studies, a helmet study in a paratrooper population, and a proposed follow-up study for prevalence and outcomes. Targets primarily adults who are hospitalized or receive health care in emergency departments and out-patient departments in the military and VA systems. Hospital discharge, ED, and outpatient data are used to identify cases of TBI (including MTBI). Routine analysis of the DVHIP registry data will cost $100,000 to $150,000 per year.

Strengths: Military- and VA-based. Military- and VA-representative. Timely. Economical. Contains baseline data (i.e., prior to injury), such as drug use and prior medical history. Includes ED data. Reports unduplicated cases; thus, allowing for study of MTBI incidence. Military cases generally healthy pre-injury. Excellent potential to follow-up adults with MTBI to characterize outcomes and the natural history of this condition; no costs for this option have been determined at this time. Includes wartime injuries. Uses International Classification of Diseases, Ninth Revision, Clinical Modification (ICD-9-CM) rubrics to code medical diagnoses.

Limitations: Does not represent the entire U.S. population. In general, younger adult males are over-represented in this database, consistent with TBI in the general population. Population in the VA system is older than the U.S. population as a whole.

Recommendations: Collaborative routine analysis with DVHIP to assess incidence, risk factors, external causes, service needs and use, and long-term consequences of MTBI and its associated disabilities in the military system. Excellent option for implementing follow-up and tracking systems for persons with MTBI (through personal interviews and medical record reviews). Because military hospitals serve enlisted personnel and their families, children constitute a small proportion of the population in these databases. Any proposed, large follow-up study would target mainly adults; findings for non-wartime injuries can be extrapolated to the general population. Special follow-up studies that target children can be proposed. Follow-up studies will allow for the characterization of the natural history of MTBI among adults. No costs have been determined for the use of these resources at this point.

NOTES

NOTES

www.ingramcontent.com/pod-product-compliance
Lightning Source LLC
Chambersburg PA
CBHW081904170526
45167CB00007B/3140